Energy, Endurance, Empowerment

Michele C. Foster

Copyright © 2015 Michele C Foster

ISBN:1508542201
ISBN-13:9781508542209

i

Energy, Endurance, Empowerment   Michele C. Foster

FORWARD

Michele C. Foster

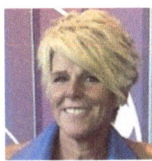 Energy is about Endurance and the Empowerment that energy provides for life's journey, both physically and financially. I am so grateful for every aspect of my life. Every day is filled with opportunities to learn something new and to decide how I can take these lessons and serve others. It is a fantastic ride!

Like many women all over the world, I spent a great portion of my life feeling lonely. One day I decided that I had been feeling sorry for myself long enough. I made a decision to get my life on track and spend the rest of my days empowering others to victory in their lives through their physical and financial health.

The first step was to get my own health on track by taking care of me. For a woman, taking care of herself is the most selfless thing she can do. When a woman is healthy she is a better lover, companion, friend, business person and leader. It took several years, but I did get the healthiest I have ever been emotionally, physically, and spiritually.

The second thing I did was investigate, examine, and undertake a study of the miraculous human body. I found:

ENERGY ~ ENDURANCE ~ EMPOWERMENT

I am now paying it forward.

Energy . . . the word, feeling, and/or belief of energy has been calling to me my entire life. As a child, the story often told about me was that I had a lot of energy. Lucky for me that I was given that belief system... one I choose to hold today.

In writing this book (with Kate) and sharing it with you, I intend to be precise with my wording and not take anything personally. Also, I will not make assumptions of anyone and will do my very best to communicate my heart!

Energy changes faster than we can understand – which is the power behind it . . .

I will discover, and share with you, things as important as:

- Muscular endurance exercises

1

- Energy boosting foods

- Empowerment from the financial chains that bind us – or passive income

You see, this is a journey - it is not a destination. As I write this I experience my own paradigm shift of energy – it's that powerful, and that majestic.

Believing you have energy is great, yet, sometimes we just feel tired. This feeling is synthetic... meaning - Not Real. When you are excited to be home, but not exhausted by your day; when your energy level is consistent from sunrise to sunset; when falling asleep, staying asleep, and rising out of bed rejuvenated... that is the energy I am connected to!

The number one cause for being so tired is fatigue. Fatigue can be the result of either internal stress (a physical condition caused by illness, allergies or lack of rest), or external stress (caused by your employment, relationships, or financial hardship).

In the next few chapters we are going to discuss the different causes of fatigue - both internal and external. And we are going to talk about solutions for fighting fatigue, including: diet, nutrition, exercise, meditation, and laughter.

.

***Disclosure: Michele C. Foster is not a medical doctor. Anyone experiencing any of these symptoms needs to visit their MD. There are NO medical claims being made in this book

Contents

1 - TYPES OF FATIGUE

Fatigue describes a lack of energy and motivation (not the sleepy feeling). Fatigue is a symptom that might not have a mental cause.

Example: Starting a new project is tiring and causes physical fatigue, resulting in the possible loss of muscle strength after simple repetitive movements.

"Normal" people who have intense physical or mental challenges can become fatigued due to:

Lack of sleep
Eating too little
Anemia
Underactive Thyroid
Chronic Fatigue Syndrome
Sleep Apnea
Urinary Tract Infection
Food Intolerance
Diabetes
Heart Disease
Depression
Glandular Fever

***Source: Boots Web MD

Abnormal Types of Fatigue:

Adrenal Fatigue - overstressed adrenal glands intensifying symptoms of hormone imbalance.

Chronic inflammation – of the ten leading causes of MORTALITY in the United States, **chronic, low-level inflammation** contributes to the pathogenesis of at least seven. These include: **heart disease, cancer, chronic lower respiratory disease, stroke, Alzheimer's disease, diabetes**, and **nephritis**.

***(Centers for Disease Control and Prevention 2011; Bastard et al. 2006; Cao 2011, Jha et al. 2009; Ferrucci et al. 2010; Glorieux et al. 2009; Kundu et al. 2008; Murphy 2012; Singh et al. 2011).*

Food allergies – A FOOD ALLERGY is an adverse immune response to a food protein. It is distinct from other adverse responses to food, such as a food intolerance.

Chemical sensitivities - multiple chemical sensitivities (MCS) are a **chronic medical condition** characterized by **symptoms** that the affected person attributes to low-level chemical exposure. Commonly accused substances include smoke, pesticides, plastics, synthetic fabrics, scented products, petroleum products, and paint fumes. Symptoms are often **vague** and **non-specific**, such as **nausea, fatigue, dizziness** and **headaches**, but also commonly include **inflammation of skin, joints, gastrointestinal tract** and **airways**.

****Source: Web MD*

12 more common types of Fatigue:

1. Lethargic – sluggish and apathetic
2. Listless – lack of interest, energy and spirit
3. Lack of Energy – mental or emotional strain
4. Tired – in need of sleep
5. Worn out – exhausted, spent
6. Weary – cause to become tired
7. Exhausted- emptied of one's physical or mental resources
8. Malaise – feeling of discomfort, illness
9. Feeling run down - iron deficiency, post menopause
10. Lack of motivation – feeling overwhelmed
11. Tires easily – constant fatigue
12. Mental fatigue – concentration and memory burnout

2 - ADAPTOGEN HERBS

We all have a finite amount of **energy** and reserves. When they are taxed, either physically or mentally, or, (more commonly) both, we experience fatigue.

Fatigue is a sign that we need to stop and recharge our batteries. If your instinct is that you are just rundown, or you are going through a period of stress in your life, you can support your body by saying no to extra activities and long hours, by ensuring you sleep well, and by using adaptogenic herbs.

What are Adaptogens?

Adaptogens are unique herbs and botanicals that strengthen the body's capacity to resist and reduce stress. They promote physical and mental performance, and normalize the body's defences.

"Adaptogenic substances are stated to have the capacity to normalize body functions and strengthen systems compromised by stress. They are reported to have a protective effect on health against a wide variety of environmental assaults."– European Medicines Agency

To be considered an Adaptogen, a plant must meet three criteria:

1. Be safe; pass testing for toxicity
2. Reduce harmful effects of stress
3. Help improve physical performance and endurance

Nature's Response to Fatigue

Adaptogenic herbs are best suited to those whose fatigue is either caused by stress, or is causing stress in their lives.

Adaptogens - or adaptogenic plants and herbs - result in the stabilization of physiological processes and the promotion of homeostasis. An example is decreased cellular sensitivity to stress.

Here is a list of important adaptogens:

- **Eleuthero root** reduces feelings of fatigue and increases resistance to low-oxygen situations, such as high altitudes and deep sea diving.
- **Schizandra** increases feelings of general well-being, and improves accuracy at work; decreases sleepiness and other symptoms of fatigue.
- **Rhodiola** reduces symptoms of fatigue and/or insomnia; improved levels of attention to detail, emotional stability, and self-esteem.
- **Wolfberry** (*Lycium barbarum)* acts as an antioxidant and adaptogen, helping to maintain good health; increase mental function and physical performance.
- **Ashwagandha** *(Withania somnifera*) acts as an antioxidant for the maintenance of good health; stimulates liver detoxification, it increases the body's resistance to stress, and may support the brain and immune function.

- **Bacopa** (*Bacopa monnieri*) acts as an antioxidant in the maintenance of brain health; has been found to be helpful for maintaining normal memory and cognitive function.

NOTE: Adaptogens can be found online. However you need to talk with your healthcare provider if you take any medications. These herbs may interact with prescription drugs.

Recent studies suggest that better management and minimization of stress support graceful aging.

In the August 2011 issue of *Nature,* a clinical study discovered that mice chronically infused with adrenaline (the stress hormone) showed results consistent with injured DNA. This might explain why humans subjected to chronic psychological stress have shorter telomeres.

*NOTE: **Telomeres** are the caps at the end of each strand of DNA; they protect our chromosomes, like the plastic tips at the end of shoelaces.*

Currently, there are studies being conducted to explore ways to combat stress and the ill effects stress has on cells and their telomeres.

Adaptogens, in supplement form, could be the solution to fighting the effects of stress, supporting healthier aging, and increased longevity.

3 - HISTORY OF ADAPTOGENS

A early definition of Adaptogens describes them as - non-specific remedies "that cause resistance to a spectrum of harmful (stressors) of different physical, chemical, and biological natures".   ***Source: huffington post*

This definition has been updated. Today adaptogens are conceptualized as a "new class of metabolic regulators (of a natural origin) which increase the ability of an organism to adapt to environmental factors and to avoid damage to such factors".

An extensive amount of research was conducted in the USSR. By 1984 more than 1,500 pharmacological and clinical studies have been published.

Adaptogens have been described as "medicine for healthy people". In 1998, the term adaptogen was allowed as a functional claim for certain products by the US Food and Drug Administration and the European Medicines Agency. The concept of adaptogen is sufficient to be considered in the assessment of traditional medicinal products.

Adaptogens in other Cultures

The concept of adaptogens as "medicine for the healthy", or in helping the body cope with stress, is a great deal similar to many remedies common in Chinese herbology, as well as other forms of traditional medicine.

Adaptogens vs. Stimulants

In spite of the theoretical normalizing effect, certain drug dosing regimens of supposed adaptogenic plant extracts are claimed to have stimulating effects on the central nervous system.

Plant adaptogens are said to stimulate the nervous system by mechanisms that are totally different from those of conventional stimulants as associated with metabolic regulation of various elements of the stress system and modulation of stimulant-response comply. Adaptogens are also claimed to be efficacious in the treatment anxiety disorder.

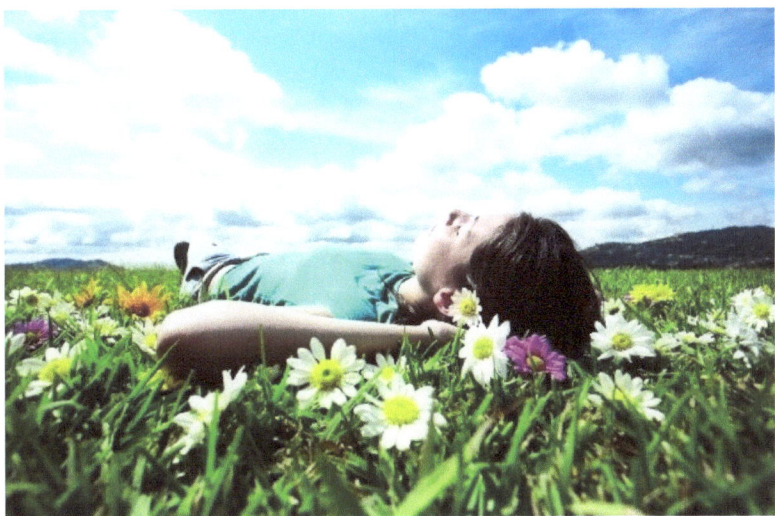

We live in a high-pressure environment. Stress from relationships, finances and careers can pile up. Before you know it, you live in a state of chronic stress. This wreaks havoc on your health, and, your mental and physical performance.

Fortunately, adaptogens, nutritional cleansing and living a healthy lifestyle are solutions to help you to stay calm, relieve stress, and unwind.

Who needs Adaptogens?

Given the calming stress relief that comes from adaptogens, the real question becomes, "Who *doesn't* need them?" When one's day is dominated by job, traffic, bills… we could all benefit from adaptogens.

Not all stress is bad, mind you. The purpose of stress is to help you react quickly in dangerous situations. The chemicals that cause stress are supposed to help the human body in quick bursts, then dissipate once a crisis is over. They aren't supposed to stay in your system for hours at a time, as they do with chronic stress.

The Symptoms of Stress

- Weight gain, or dramatic weight loss
- Hair loss
- Regular headaches
- Immune system suppression
- Digestive issues

4 - PHARMACODYNAMICS

The action mechanism of adaptogens has been hard to rationalize. However, by 1965 it had been demonstrated that the adaptogenic effect is a dependent cellular transaction.

***Reference Breckman 1969 "New Substances of Plant Origin that Increases Non specific Resistance"

By 1980, it was clear that the adaptogens effects operate on the sympathetic nervous system.

What are the Sympathetic and Parasympathetic Nervous Systems?

The **sympathetic nervous system** mediates sexual arousal, reaction to emergencies, and vigilance by increasing your heart rate, boosting your blood pressure, and speeding up your breathing. It is responsible for the classic "fight or flight" response, which is mediated by the two main chemical messengers epinephrine (adrenaline) and norepinephrine (noradrenaline).

Over stimulation of the sympathetic nervous system can lead to anxiety, hypertension, and digestive disturbances.

The **parasympathetic nervous system**, in contrast, primarily counters the sympathetic one by mediating the body's calming and relaxing functions. If you meditate, eat a big meal, take a nap… the parasympathetic nervous system kicks in, slowing down your heart rate.

Overstimulation of the parasympathetic nervous system can result in low blood pressure and fatigue.

When they work in conjunction, these two systems (the sympathetic and parasympathetic) work great. Problems occur when the two systems are out of balance.

***Source: Laura Berman Ph

This is a subject near and dear to Michele and what follows is her own story of toxic overload…

> "Back in the early 1990's, I was living in Seattle, Washington. I was getting treatment from a natural health care practitioner there, that measured toxicity."

> "I was diagnosed with "massive" amounts of mercury in my body which could be fatal if not removed. They believed that the mercury came from a dentist using amalgam fillings in my teeth when I had many cavities as a teenager."

> "The health care practitioner used a process called Chelation, which I believe to be the only natural solution to this issue. After I completed 17 of the suggested 20 treatments, I was at a "safe" level."

> "That was the beginning of my awareness of the effect of toxicity in the body. The process of removing that toxicity was brutal, yet the end outcome was life-changing to my health."

> "I believe the body cannot function correctly with the increased amounts of toxicity in our world. Since that time back in the 1990's when my body was detoxified - environmental toxicity levels have

increased dramatically."

"My concern over toxicity levels in the body led me to become a certified nutritionist and practitioner in the energy medicine field. I am also a magnetic therapist, and in that capacity I work with the natural electromagnetic fields in the body and the world around us. I am not a medical doctor."

5 - TOXINS

Toxins in our everyday life ~

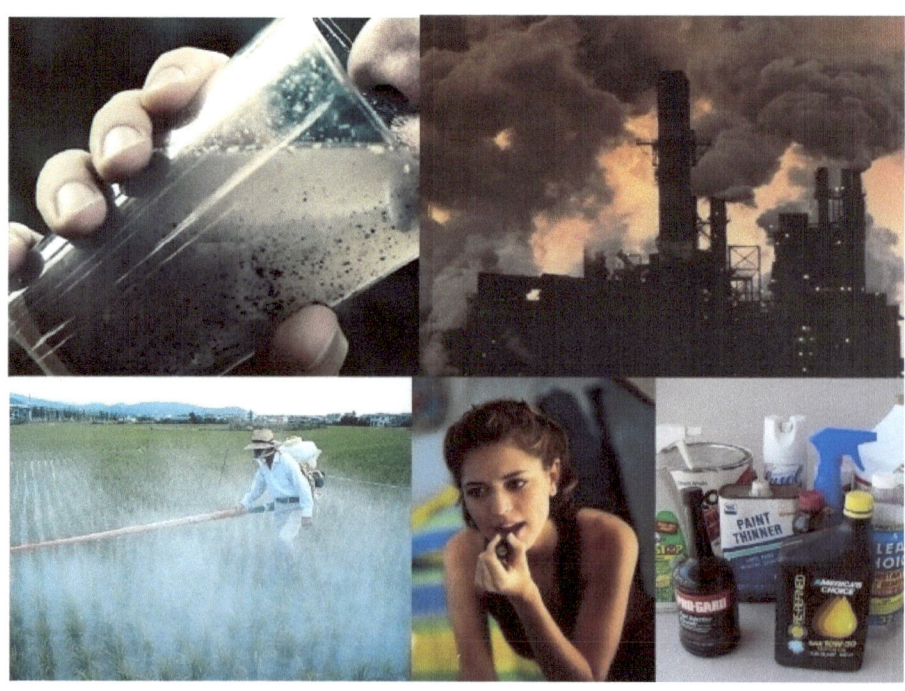

The term "**environmental toxins**" can sometimes explicitly include synthetic contaminants such as industrial pollutants and other artificially made toxic substances.

Toxins can be small molecules, peptides, or proteins that are capable of causing disease on contact through absorption by body tissues interacting with biological macromolecules such as enzymes or cellular receptors. Toxins vary greatly in their severity, ranging from minor and acute (as a bee sting) to almost immediately deadly (as in botullinum toxin).

Toxicity is the degree to which a substance can damage an organism. Toxicity can refer to the whole organism, such as animal, bacterium, or plant. It can also refer to the effect on a substructure of the organism, such as a cell, or an organ (i.e. the liver).

Top signs you may be suffering from a buildup of toxicity:

- Sugar cravings
- Low or inconsistent energy
- Bloating or gas
- Caffeine addiction
- Binge eating or drinking
- Mood swings
- Irritable anxiety
- Brain fog or difficulty concentrating
- Fluid retention
- Migraines or headaches

6 - NUTRITIONAL CLEANSING

What is Nutritional Cleansing? It is the process of flooding your body with rich nutrients, while gently cleansing the impurities away.

Why do Nutritional Cleansing? Because of toxic overload to our bodies. Just the environmental toxins we are fighting against to stay healthy are staggering - over 250 known to date, while 20 years ago they were non existent.

If 2009, UCLA did a study of 1000 newborn babies. Testing these babies showed that over 900 had jet fuel oil in their little bodies.

We are not suggesting a fad diet detox. Juice cleanses and body purifying diets have become very popular in recent years. While there are a host of benefits to cleaning up your diet and focusing on healthier foods, many diet detoxes, or cleanses, are unsafe and unhealthy.

Health professionals warn that these fad diet products can be dangerous (especially if followed for a long period of time). They can lead to muscle breakdown, electrolyte imbalances, and nutrient deficiencies.

Additionally, much of the weight lost on these programs is water weight, not fat. Once you discontinue the cleanse and go back to normal eating, it's common to regain the weight that was lost."

Solutions?

You could live in a bubble and isolate yourself from the environment and ordinary activities of life.

Or you could practice **whole body nutritional cleansing**.

Whatever you decide to do, it must be doable, non invasive, and most of all, have proven results.

A Nutritional Cleansing Diet includes:

1. **Fiber rich foods** - Fruits and vegetables rich in vitamins, minerals, antioxidants, and fiber. Adding a lot of fruits and vegetables can provide you with adequate natural fiber to help provide your body with cleansing benefits.

2. **Eat dark greens daily** - Eating at least 1-2 servings dark greens each day can help support your nutritional cleanse by providing a lot of fiber, antioxidants and other nutrients.

3. **Eat unprocessed, whole grains** - 100% whole grains are another great nutrient-rich food group. They contain protein, vitamins and are also a good source of fiber. If you're interested in a cleanse and improving your diet, switch your grain choices to 100% whole grain.

4. **Choose lean protein at each meal** - Many nutritional cleanses focus mainly on fruits and vegetables. Although this has many benefits, it's important to also include sources of lean protein at each meal.

5. **Ditch processed foods** - Avoid foods that are highly refined and highly processed such as: candy and sweets; processed meats like bologna, sausage or bacon, snack cakes and pastries; cereals, frozen meals, chips and crackers.

6. **Drink a lot of fluids** - One very important part of a healthy diet and a nutritional cleanse is ensuring that you consume an adequate amount of clear, sugar-free, caffeine-free fluids. Your body needs these fluids each day to stay hydrated and to function properly.

A Nutritional Cleansing Lifestyle includes:

1. **An appointment with your doctor.** Before making any large dietary or lifestyle changes, it's important to check in with your doctor. Talk about your desire for weight loss and the use of a nutritional cleanse to help reach your goal.

2. **Take a probiotic supplement.** Like fermented foods, probiotic supplements may help improve your digestion and reduce minor digestive issues (like constipation or bloating).

3. **Take fiber supplements.** Adequate fiber is important to a healthy diet. In addition, fiber can help support a nutritional cleanse by improving bowel health.

4. **Exercise regularly.** Consistent and regular physical activity is a complimentary part of weight loss. Add exercise to help quicken weight loss with your nutritional cleanse. Aim for at least 150 minutes of aerobic activity each week, including 40 minutes of strength training. Also consider adding in - relaxing, cleansing exercises like yoga or tai chi. These are a great way of adding beneficial activity and supporting a cleansing diet and lifestyle.

5. **Sleep 7-9 hours nightly.** Adequate rest each night is important to your overall health. In addition, sleeping the recommended 7-9 hours nightly can help support a healthy weight and weight loss.

Results! **Energy ~ Endurance ~ Empowerment**

Source: http://www.wikihow.com/Lose-Weight-With-Nutritional-Cleansing

7 - TEN STEPS TO ENDURANCE

#1. Whole Body Nutritional Cleansing

Nutritional Cleansing helps give your body the nutrition it needs to cleanse itself naturally. It's designed to feed and nourish your body (unlike other "cleanses" that deplete your body through laxatives or diuretics). It helps the body better cope with stress and supports improved mental and physical performance and overall health.

#2. Daily Doses of Adaptogens – "Medicine for the Healthy"

AM to PM – all day, every day. Plant-based adaptogens are perfect for combating the effects of stress and fatigue. Adaptogens are a powerful asset for building endurance and improving overall personal performance.

#3. Meditation

15 minutes, 2 times daily - use a quiet process of counting down from 100 to 0. Taking 4-second inhales and exhales, focus your mind on what you want in life, from the material, to the spiritual, to the emotional.

Meditation often involves an internal effort to self-regulate the mind in some way. Meditation is also used to clear the mind and ease many health issues, such as high **blood pressure, depression,** and **anxiety.**

#4. Get Plenty of Rest

You need 7-9 hours of quality sleep every nigh. Sleepiness causes accidents, "dumbs" you down, and, can lead to serious health issues such as:

- Heart disease
- Heart attack
- Heart failure
- Irregular heartbeat
- High blood pressure
- Stroke
- Diabetes

 According to some estimates, 90% of people with insomnia - a sleep disorder characterized by having trouble falling asleep and staying asleep - also have another health condition. Sleep specialists say that sleep-deprived men and women report lower libidos and less interest in sex. Depleted energy, sleepiness, and increased tension may be largely to blame.

#5. Daily Exercise

Aerobic Exercise – We need at least 150 minutes of aerobic activity each week; walking, jogging/running, swimming, or cycling.

Resistance Exercise – We need at least 40 minutes of resistance training each week. This strengthens your muscles by carrying a load to build up your arms, legs, core, and more. This is referred to as muscular endurance exercises.

Resistance training is important because of its role in building and maintaining muscle. You truly will lose it if you don't use it; to stave off muscle decline, you must carry a load. Maintaining and building muscle is good for your metabolism, makes you strong, prevents falling, prevents injury, and lifts your mood.

#6. Focus on Nutrition

Nutrition is 85% of the health equation – a proper mix of proteins, low glycemic carbohydrates and fats 3 times a day, along with healthy snacking every 2 hours. Nutrition is the baseline for Health. Your Body is a Miracle – put the right things in it and the right things happen… FAST!!

#7. Decrease Stress

Mental and physical stress
Stress triggers higher levels of the hormone, cortisol. Cortisol regulates a number of important functions including immune response.

Recommendations - to decrease stress practice yoga, exercise and use other relaxation techniques.

Next time you're stressed out, you might just grab someone you love for a cuddle session! The hormone oxytocin is known to curb the body's stress response -- it's not called the "**cuddle hormone**" without reason. Our bodies release oxytocin when we experience positive interactions with others.

Oxytocin "helps your blood vessels relax and even regenerates the heart from stress-related damage." ***Source: Huffington Post*

#8. Organic Foods

Organic foods are "clean", meaning they lack chemicals. When foods with chemicals are eaten, your body has to process out those toxins. So by eating clean, organic food, you are that much ahead of the process to a healthier functioning body.

Organic foods are labelled as such and can be found at stores such as Whole Foods, Trader Joes and Costco. You can also buy sprays to clean the vegetables and fruits of chemicals. However, we believe it is easier to just buy organic foods.

The worst foods to buy and eat are non-organic lemons and limes, corn, grain fed chickens and cows. All of these products are poisoned with herbicides, pesticides and steroids, and cause your body to become acidic.

#9. Acidic vs Alkaline

In **chemistry**, pH is a measure of the **acidity** or **basicity** of an **aqueous solution**.

The abbreviation pH stands for 'power' of 'Hydrogen'. It means the concentration of hydrogen ions in a solution.

Solutions with a pH less than 7 are said to be **acidic**, and solutions with a pH greater than 7 are **basic** or **alkaline**. Pure water has a pH very close to 7.

Acidic bodies carry inflammation. Inflammation is the body's attempt at self-protection; the aim being to remove harmful stimuli - including damaged cells, irritants, or pathogens - and begin the healing process.

The word inflammation comes from the Latin "inflammo", meaning "I set alight, I ignite".

Eating an Alkaline Diet:

- Increases power, strength, and energy levels
- Increases the blood's ability to carry more oxygen = more endurance and power
- Provides natural buffers to help clear out excessive acid production

- Reduces illness, chronic fatigue, fibromyalgia, cancers
- Promotes weight loss
- Enhances hydration

***Source: Dr. Paul Biandoch

Your blood is designed to work best in the alkaline range, and tries to maintain it at all times.

Our ancient diet, before the start of agriculture, was alkaline based. Our blood functions best at an alkaline pH of 7.35-7.45. This design is built into our DNA. Blood can carry its full load of oxygen only at this range of pH.

Once the blood drops below a pH of 7.0 it becomes acidic. Its oxygen capacity then declines; along with the loss of oxygen, the blood's capacity to detoxify declines.

***Source: Colgan Institute 2010

> *NOTE: Michele says - In my quest to alkalize my body and to "balance" myself, I tried many things. The foods listed below are powerful tools used in the fight to alkalize the body, and are the same foods recommended by John Anderson, who is affectionately called the "mineral man".*

Products recommended to get our bodies alkaline are:
- Greens Supplements
- Alkaline water
- Non-Carbonated mineral rich water
- Fresh lemon water in the morning
- Organic Dark roast coffee

#10. Live Love Laugh– Being happy and having an 'attitude of gratitude' is a decision you make every day. Put 'happy' and 'gratitude' on your calendar, making sure that you spend time with family and friends. Take time to laugh . . . either hang out with people that make you laugh, rent funny movies or listen to a comedian. Just laugh until you have tears in your eyes.

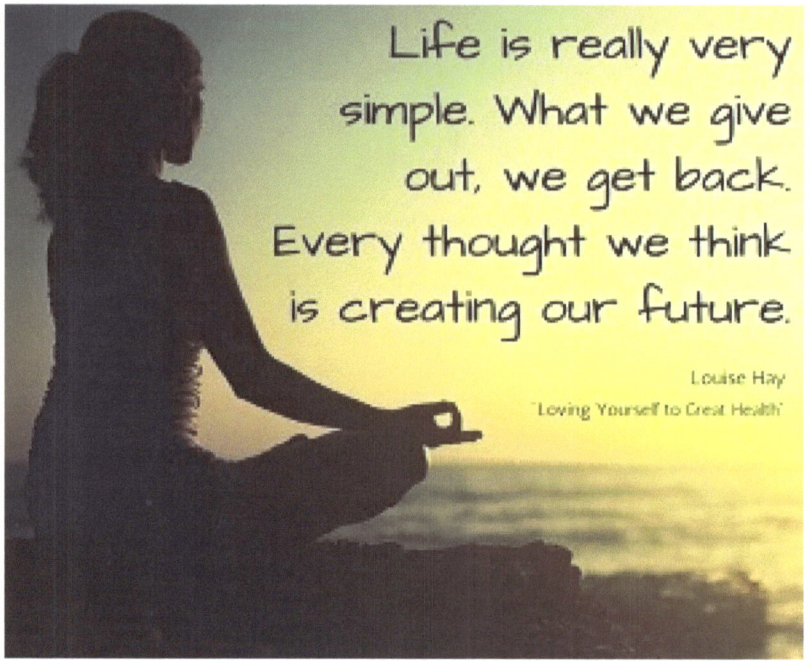

Life is really very simple. What we give out, we get back. Every thought we think is creating our future.

Louise Hay
"Loving Yourself to Great Health"

8 - CASE STUDIES

Case Study #1

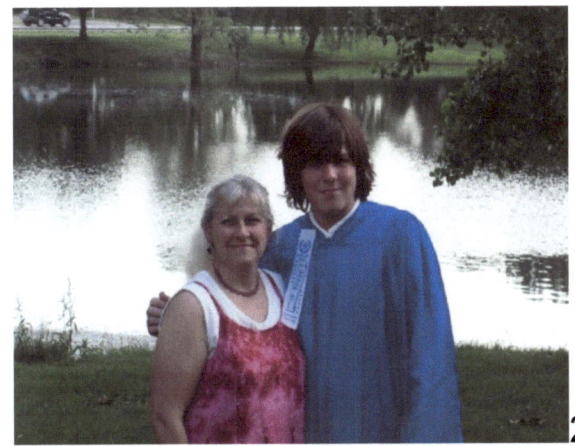

2005

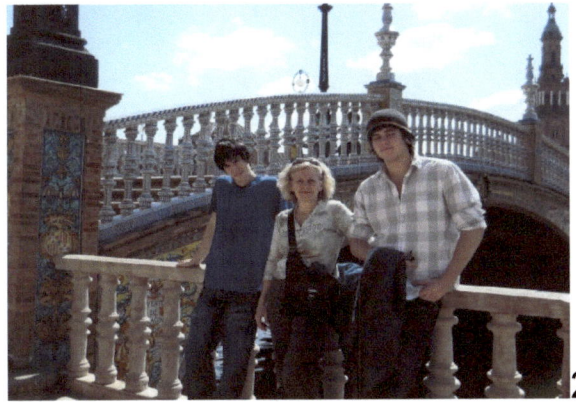

2012

Claire S. Story - Claire is a nutritionist, and has always cooked nutritious meals for her family, 3 times a day. Her son David was anaphylactic as a baby and young boy, so she had to check every ingredient that he was consuming.

Claire suffered with overweight her entire life. If fact, the 2005 picture was taken while she was doing Weight Watchers, and she says it was the best of the best – till it wasn't anymore.

Then Claire started doing nutritional cleansing and practicing a healthy lifestyle. Her body released 22 inches. To date she has maintained this body reduction while maintaining her regimen of adaptogens, proteins, and nutritional cleansing.

Case Study #2

Labor Day 2013   December 12th, 2013 minus 45lbs

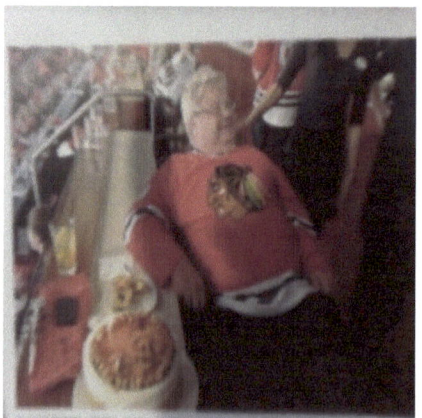
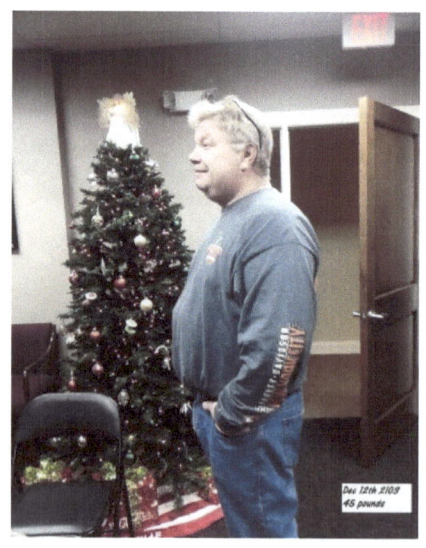

Tim S. Story: Tim practiced the nutritional cleansing lifestyle for 4 months. He lost 45 pounds with minimal exercise.

Case Study #3

Michele Foster's Story: Before Michele started nutritional cleansing and practicing a healthy lifestyle, she felt good, but not great. She believed that she had a lot of energy, and at the same time, believed she was getting more and more sick each year.

Michele was asked to look at information about a nutritional cleansing product by one of the patients in the clinic where she worked.

Molly, a good friend of one of the doctors, asked Michele to listen to a CD by a nutritionist. She did, and the CD captured her interest because of the information about whole body nutritional cleansing at the cellular level (ie: remembering her chelation).

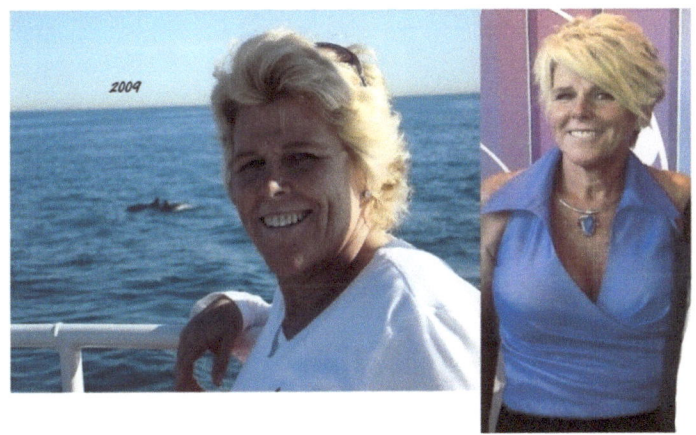

Since then, she has practiced a nutritional cleansing lifestyle, and has released 23 pounds and 21 inches.

Michele says: "I feel amazing and have more sustainable focused energy than I have ever had in my life! It has been 6 years now. I believe in the nutritional cleansing lifestyle. Flushing out the toxins, flooding the body with dense nutrition, reducing stress levels, and lengthening my telomeres is a game changer!"

9 - EMPOWERMENT

Energy is about Endurance and the Empowerment that energy provides for life's journey, both physically and financially.

Empowerment is about your financial journey. When it is YOUR life, YOUR way, when you are in control of YOUR lifestyle choices... that is when purpose-filled work becomes meaningful. And it doesn't even seem like work!

Before, coming from a corporate environment, I did not understand what a passive income could mean. I even feared the boredom of not having a job, and, I was even a little scared of the idea of quitting my job – To what? For what? With what?

I knew that the stress of the work I was doing was killing me, and people around us. I knew that year after year of living with the stress would be hard to sustain. So I decided to explore the idea of passive income and see how it could improve the quality of my life.

With a driven personality and a sense of urgency, both of us, I was motivated to explore what it means to be an entrepreneur.

Empowerment means to live… FULL TIME, to feel joy… FULL TIME, and to have purpose… FULL TIME.

> Michele says, "The purpose I longed to find I now know is - service to others. I have this purpose without the need for approval, or a paycheck, or someone giving me permission to live, or to make a living, or end it. This has been the most empowering realization. I am living this realization constantly, at a deeper and deeper level.
>
> The more people I serve - the deeper my purpose and self-fulfillment. The more financially secure I am - the more I explore my true desires, beliefs, and joys."

Pursuing a passive income is at times challenging and always exciting. It has been a mission and a destination that continues to drive Michele farther than I ever dreamed.

The level of energy that I have attained from proper nutrition and a healthy lifestyle, has empowered me to reach for my dreams; to serve on a playing field that is only for the willing… to do what others won't so I can have and be what others can't.

What makes that okay to say is that anyone can experience for themselves this empowerment and the freedom it provides. And, anyone can join me on this journey to experience energy, endurance, and empowerment… to achieve true freedom.

I am experiencing this freedom for the first time in my 50's. Friends of mine are experiencing this freedom in their 20's, 30's, 40's and even into their 80's. This freedom is here for anyone and everyone who can capture the vision.

Energy ~ Endurance ~ Empowerment ~ Very cool!

For more information visit: http://askmicheletoday.com and

Contact Michele Foster at askmicheletoday@gmail.com

PH: 847.323.2419

GLOSSARY

Fatigue / stress: the number one cause of disease in the body. Whether it is chronic (constant), physical, mental, or adrenal fatigue, there are nature's answers to stress and better personal performance.

Adaptogens are unique plants that strengthen the body's capacity to resist and reduce stress, as well as promote physical and mental performance. Whether you need a high energy pick-me-up, an ally in your fight against chronic stress, or natural support for today's overtaxed immune systems, you will find solutions to these problems in this book.

Pharmacodynamics is the study of the biochemical and physiological effect of drugs on the body or on microorganisms, or on parasites within, or on the body and the mechanisms of drug reaction – what the drug does to the body.

Toxicity There are 34,000 pesticides and herbicides registered with the Environmental Protection Agency (EPA), plus about 66,000 commercial chemicals. Of these 100,000 toxins, the United States uses about one-quarter of the volume of all of them that are used in the world each year. They are everywhere, all around us, every day. Research shows that the average person's body now contains between 40 and 80 different chemical residues at toxic levels. These chemicals are stored defensively in our fat cells under the skin, and throughout the fats in our liver and kidneys, and in our thyroid and adrenal glands. They are especially toxic when they accumulate in the fatty tissue that comprises most of our brain and spinal cord.

***Source - Colgan Institute 201

35

www.ingramcontent.com/pod-product-compliance
Lightning Source LLC
Chambersburg PA
CBHW050756290526
45792CB00008B/2210